Understanding Asthma

MANAGING AND

MINIMIZINGTHE IMPACT OF

ASTHMA ON INDIVIDUALS

AND SOCIETY.

by Taylor jones

TAYLOR JONES

TABLE OF CONTENT

TAYLOR JONES

TAYLOR JONES

Introduction

Asthma is a constant respiratory condition that influences a large number of individuals around the world. A complex and possibly weakening illness causes irritation and limiting of the aviation routes, prompting breathing troubles. Asthma can appear in different structures and seriousness levels, making it urgent to have a complete comprehension of this condition and its administration.

As of late, the pervasiveness of asthma has been on the ascent, influencing individuals of any age, sexes, and identities. It is assessed that north of 300 million people overall right now experience the ill effects of asthma, and this number is projected to increment before long. With such a critical effect on general wellbeing, it is indispensable to dive into the complexities of asthma to all the more likely grasp its causes, side effects, triggers, and accessible treatment choices.

Understanding asthma requires investigating its fundamental instruments. Asthma is essentially described by the aggravation of the aviation routes, prompting their extreme touchiness and resulting restricting. This irritation can be set off by different elements, including allergens (like residue parasites, dust, or pet dander), respiratory contaminations, work out, cool air, and certain meds.

Therefore, people with asthma frequently experience intermittent episodes of wheezing, hacking, chest snugness, and windedness.

To successfully oversee asthma, it is fundamental to recognize and grasp its side effects. By perceiving the early indications of an asthma assault, people can make a suitable move to keep the condition from declining.

Legitimate conclusion of asthma includes assessing a singular's clinical history, leading lung capability tests, and surveying their reaction to bronchodilators.

Moreover, figuring out the triggers that can incite asthma side effects is critical for forestalling assaults and dealing with the condition really. Ecological elements, like openness to allergens or air contamination, can assume a huge part in setting off asthma side effects. By recognizing and staying away from these triggers, people with asthma can diminish the recurrence and seriousness of their side effects.

While there is right now no solution for asthma, there are different treatment choices accessible to control the side effects and work on the personal satisfaction for people with this condition. Meds, including bronchodilators and mitigating drugs, are usually recommended to oversee asthma side effects and decrease aviation route aggravation. Moreover, fostering an asthma activity plan with the direction of medical care experts can assist people with observing their condition and answer suitably during asthma assaults.

Asthma

Bronchial asthma (or asthma) is a lung illness.

Your aviation routes get restricted and enlarged and are impeded by overabundance bodily fluid.

Drugs can treat these side effects.

Asthma, likewise called bronchial asthma, is a sickness that influences your lungs. It's an ongoing (progressing) condition, meaning it doesn't go away and needs progressing clinical the executives.

Asthma influences in excess of 25 million individuals in the U.S. at present. This absolute incorporates more

than 5 million youngsters. Asthma can be perilous on the off chance that you don't seek treatment.

What is an asthma assault?

At the point when you inhale regularly, muscles around your aviation routes are loose, allowing air to move

effectively and discreetly. During an asthma assault,

three things can occur:

Bronchospasm: The muscles around the aviation routes contract (fix). At the point when they fix, it makes your aviation routes limited.

Air can't stream uninhibitedly through

contracted aviation routes.

Irritation: The coating of your aviation routes becomes enlarged.

Enlarged aviation routes don't let as much air in or out of your lungs.

Bodily fluid creation: During the assault, your body makes more bodily fluid. This thick bodily fluid obstructs aviation routes.

At the point when your aviation routes get tighter, you make a sound called wheezing when you inhale, a clamor your aviation routes make when you inhale out. You could likewise hear an asthma assault

hit a fuel or an eruption. It's the term for when your asthma isn't controlled.

Types Of Asthma

Asthma is separated into types in light of the reason and the seriousness of side effects.

Medical care suppliers distinguish asthma as:

1. Discontinuous: This kind of asthma travels every which way so you can feel ordinary in between asthma flares.

2. Persi/stent: Steady asthma implies you have side effects a significant part of the time.

Side effects can be gentle, moderate or serious. Medical services suppliers base asthma seriousness on how frequently you have side effects.

They likewise consider how well you can get things done during an assault.

Asthma has various causes:

3. Hypersensitive: Certain individuals' sensitivities can

cause an asthma assault. Allergens incorporate things like molds, dusts and pet

dander.

4.Non-unfavorably susceptible: Outside variables can cause

asthma to erupt. Work out, stress, disease and weather conditions might cause a flare.

5. Grown-up beginning: This kind of asthma begins after the age of 18.

Pediatric: Additionally called youth

asthma,

this sort of asthma frequently starts previously

the age of 5, and can happen in babies and

little children. Youngsters might grow out of asthma.

You ought to ensure that you talk about it with your supplier before you choose whether your kid needs to have an inhaler accessible in the event that they have an asthma assault. Your kid's medical care supplier can assist you with understanding the gambles.

6. Work out incited asthma: This type is set off by practice and is additionally called work out instigated bronchospasm. Word related asthma: This kind of

asthma happens essentially to individuals who work around aggravating substances. Asthma-COPD cross-over disorder

7. (ACOS): This type happens when you have both asthma and constant obstructive pneumonic illness (COPD). The two infections make it challenging to relax.

Who can get asthma?

Anybody can foster asthma at whatever stage in life.

Individuals with sensitivities or individuals presented to tobacco smoke are bound to foster asthma.

This incorporates handed-down cigarette smoke

(openness to another person who is smoking) and thirdhand smoke (openness to attire or surfaces where some has smoked).

Insights show that individuals appointed female upon entering the world will generally have asthma more than individuals allocated male upon entering the world. Asthma influences Individuals of color more habitually than different races.

SYMPTOMS AND CAUSES

Specialists don't have the foggiest idea why certain individuals have asthma while others don't. Yet, certain elements present a higher gamble:

(I) Sensitivities: Having sensitivities can

raise your gamble of creating asthma.

Natural variables: Individuals can foster asthma after openness to things that disturb the aviation routes.

These substances incorporate allergens, poisons, vapor and second-or third-hand smoke.

These can be particularly unsafe to babies and small kids whose invulnerable frameworks haven't wrapped up creating.

(ii) Hereditary qualities: In the event that your family has a background marked by asthma or unfavorably susceptible illnesses, you have a higher gamble of fostering the sickness.

(iii) Respiratory infection

Certain respiratory contaminations, for example, respiratory syncytial infection (RSV), can harm small kids' creating lungs.

Common Asthma Attack

You can have an asthma assault assuming you interact with substances that bother you.

Medical care suppliers refer to these substances as "triggers." Understanding what sets off your asthma makes it simpler to keep away from asthma assaults.

For certain individuals, a trigger can welcome on an assault immediately. For others, or at different times, an assault might begin hours or days after the fact.

Triggers can be different for every individual. In any case, a few normal triggers include:

<u>Air contamination:</u>

Numerous things outside can cause an asthma assault.

Air contamination incorporates plant emanations, vehicle exhaust, fierce blaze smoke and the sky is the limit from there.

Dust parasites: You can't see these bugs; however, they are in our homes.

In the event that you have a residue

Parasite sensitivity, this can cause an asthma assault.

Workout: For certain individuals, working out can cause an assault.

Shape: Soggy spots can bring forth form, which can create issues in the event that you have asthma. You don't need to be oversensitive to form to have an assault.

Bothers: Cockroaches, mice and other family nuisances can cause asthma assaults.

Pets: Your pets can cause asthma assaults. On the off chance that you're susceptible to pet dander (Dried skin chips), taking in the dander can aggravate your aviation routes.

Tobacco smoke: In the event that you or somebody in your home smokes, you have a higher chance of creating asthma. You ought to never smoke in encased places like the vehicle or home, and the best arrangement is to stop smoking. Your supplier can help.

Solid synthetics or scents. These things

can set off assaults in certain individuals.

Certain word related openings. You can

be presented to numerous things at your

specific employment, counting cleaning

items, dust from flour or wood, or

different synthetic substances.

These can all be triggers assuming you

have asthma.

Different Signs and Side effects Of Asthma

Individuals with asthma normally have

self-evident

side effects. These signs and side effects

look like numerous respiratory

contaminations:

Chest snugness, agony or tension.

Hacking (particularly round evening

time).

Windedness, Wheezing.

With asthma, you might not have these side effects with each flare.

You can have various side effects and signs at various times with constant asthma.

Additionally, side effects can change between asthma assaults.

DIAGNOSIS AND TESTS

Your medical care supplier will audit your clinical history, including data about your folks and kin.

Your supplier will likewise get some information about your side effects. Your supplier should know any set of experiences of sensitivities, dermatitis (an uneven rash brought about by sensitivities) and other lung sicknesses.

Your supplier might arrange spirometry. This test estimates wind current through your lungs and is utilized to determine and screen your advancement to have treatment. Your medical services supplier might arrange a chest X-beam, blood test or skin test.

MANAGEMENT AND TREATMENT

You have choices to help deal with your asthma. Your medical services supplier may endorse prescriptions to control side effects.

These include:

1. Bronchodilators: These prescriptions loosen up the muscles around your

aviation routes, the casual muscles let the aviation routes move air.

They likewise let bodily fluid move all the more without any problem through the aviation routes. These prescriptions assuage your side effects when they occur

furthermore, are utilized for irregular and

ongoing asthma.

2. Mitigating prescriptions: These
meds diminish expanding and bodily
fluid
creation in your aviation routes.
They make it simpler for air to enter and
leave your lungs.
Your medical services supplier might
recommend them to require consistently
to control or forestall your side effects of
persistent asthma.

3. Biologic the cutlasses for asthma:
These are utilized for serious asthma
when side effects continue regardless of
legitimate inhaler treatment.
You can take asthma drugs in a few
various ways. You might take in the
drugs utilizing a metered-portion inhaler,

nebulizer or one more sort of asthma inhaler. Your medical care supplier might recommend oral drugs that you swallow.

Asthma Control

The objective of asthma treatment is to control side effects.

Asthma control implies you:

Can would the things you like to accomplish at work furthermore, home.

Have no (or insignificant) asthma side effects.

Seldom need to utilize your reliever medication (salvage inhaler).

Rest without asthma intruding on your rest.

How to screen asthma side effects?

(I) You ought to monitor your asthma

side effect. It's a significant piece of dealing with the infection.

(ii) Your medical care supplier might request to utilize a pinnacle stream (PF) meter.

This gadget estimates how quick you can blow air out of your lungs. It can assist your supplier with making acclimations to your drug. It likewise tells you on the off chance that your side effects are deteriorating.

PREVENTION

How might I forestall an asthma assault?

On the off chance that your medical services supplier says you have asthma, you'll have to sort out what triggers an assault. Keeping away from the triggers can assist you with staying away from an assault. However, you can't keep yourself from getting asthma.

LIVING WITH AN ASTHMA ACTION PLAN

What is an asthma activity plan?

Your medical services supplier will work with you to foster an asthma activity plan. This plan lets you know how and when to utilize your medications.

It likewise guides you based on your asthma side effects and when to look for crisis care.

Get some information about anything you don't have any idea.

WHAT TO DO IF YOU HAVE A SEVERE ASTHMA ATTACK?

1. On the off chance that you have an extreme asthma assault, you want to get quick clinical consideration.

The principal thing you ought to do is utilize your salvage inhaler.

A salvage inhaler utilizes effective prescriptions to open up your aviation routes.

It's not quite the same as an upkeep inhaler,

which you utilize consistently.

2. You ought to utilize the salvage inhaler when side effects are irritating

you and you can utilize it all the more as often as possible in the event that your flare is serious.

On the off chance that your salvage inhaler doesn't help or you try not to have it with you, go to the crisis division assuming that you have Uneasiness or frenzy.

Somewhat blue fingernails, pale blue lips (in light-cleaned individuals)

or dim or whitish lips or

gums (in darker looking individuals)

Chest torment or tension.

Hacking that won't stop or extreme wheezing when you relax, Trouble talking.

Pale, sweat-soaked face.

Extremely speedy or fast relaxing.

FREQUENTLY ASKED QUESTIONS

How can you say whether do or don't have asthma?

You'll have to see a medical care supplier to see whether you have asthma or another condition.

There are other respiratory illnesses that make it hard to inhale or cause hacking and wheezing.

Could asthma at any point be relieved?

No. Asthma can't be relieved, however it very well may be made due. Youngsters might grow out of asthma as they progress in years.

For what reason is my asthma more regrettable around evening time?

Asthma that deteriorates around evening time is in some cases called evening asthma or nighttime asthma.

There are no unequivocal reasons that this occurs, yet there are a few reasonable deductions.

These include:

The manner in which you rest: Dozing on your back can bring about bodily fluid dribbling into your throat or indigestion returning up from your stomach.

Additionally, dozing on your back comes down on your chest furthermore, lungs, which makes breathing more troublesome. Nonetheless, lying face down or on

your side can come down on your lungs.

Triggers in your room and triggers that occur at night: You might find your covers, sheets and pads have dust bugs, form or pet hair on them. In the event that you've been outside in the afternoon, you might have gotten dust with you.

Prescription secondary effects:

A few medications that treat asthma, like steroids and montelukast, can influence your rest.

Air that is excessively hot or excessively chilly:

Hot air can make aviation routes slender when you take in. Cold air is an asthma trigger for certain individuals.

Lung capability changes: Lung capability

diminishes around evening time as a characteristic cycle.

Asthma is ineffectively controlled during the day: Side effects that aren't controlled During the day could be worse around evening time.

It means a lot to work with your supplier to ensure your asthma side effects are controlled both constantly. Treating evening time side effects is vital.

Serious asthma assaults, and in some cases

passings, can occur around evening time.

Conclusion

All in all, understanding asthma is principal in tending to the developing pervasiveness and effect of this persistent respiratory condition. By digging into the complexities of asthma, including its causes, side effects, triggers, and treatment choices, people and medical care experts can really oversee and control this incapacitating sickness.

Asthma's fundamental aggravation and restricting of the aviation routes can bring about critical breathing challenges and   decreased personal satisfaction. Perceiving the early signs and side effects of asthma, for example, wheezing, hacking, chest snugness, and windedness, takes into consideration convenient intercession and preventive measures. Recognizing and keeping away from triggers that incite asthma side effects, for example, allergens and ecological contaminations, assumes a critical part in limiting the recurrence and seriousness of asthma assaults. By taking on a proactive methodology and making an asthma activity plan, people can oversee their condition, permitting them to participate in everyday exercises with decreased constraints.

While there is as of now no remedy for asthma, headways in clinical examination and treatment choices have essentially worked on the administration of this condition. Meds, including bronchodilators and calming drugs, give alleviation and assist with diminishing aviation route aggravation, permitting people to have more agreeable existences.

Normal checking of lung capability and reliable correspondence with medical services experts empower customized asthma the executives design that take care of individual necessities.

Moreover, bringing issues to light about asthma and giving training on its side effects, triggers, and the board is fundamental. By advancing asthma proficiency among people, families, schools, and networks, the disgrace encompassing asthma can be decreased, and fitting help can be given to those impacted.